The Healing of the Earth

Thomas Medonis

Edited With Love Through Brien Coleman

2016

An essence known as ether has hitherto existed. This immeasurable substance isn't wildly known to the populace. This etheric ocean that fills the space throughout our universe is transmitting electronic currents into your very own etheric body this very second, a body that is composed of energy threads. A contemporary definition of ether is that two organic groups attach to an oxygen atom. Minerals attached to oxygen atoms will therefore conduct energy currents. Are we a formation of wires? How can electricity flow through the air?

Ancient philosophy claimed that ether was the medium that filled space. Through the study and practice of ancient spiritual wisdom one can obtain a super sensibility toward the spiritual world that forms the ether. The pervasive imperceptible spirits throughout nature that form our earth can become visible. The mind must, however, perform a transmutation in order to develop this spiritual sense. Think of the fine roots of a plant "magnetizing in" all the essential elements within the soil for its developing form. If one is to pursue the consuming desires of form (ego), then no super-sensibility can occur. We must be reborn to join the kingdom.

A soul center dwells in every living form and emits a soul body. The soul is omnipresent and omnipotent. An indefinable essence at the root of our very existence is the mystery that makes humans what they are (I will later make the same case for the sun). A metaphor can be drawn here: that the souls evolution exists like that of the force within a seed. Soul is not the matter presented in seed form, but rather the force that will extract the living being out of the seed to fulfill its purpose in physical manifestation.

Modern physics has proven the existence of these eternal elements and their emitting rays. The proof for perpetual life on this earth is located right within the essence of every being. Everyone has soul. It all depends how far from soul awareness each individual is. The invisible force that animates the body is one of the three main bodies which form mans physique, the physical body and the eternal soul being the other two.

In other words, without certain invisible omnipresent forces man could not exist in the physical form. No living being could. The great separation between man and animal, who both house soul, is the great power conducted by the higher mind. It actually takes more energy to generate thought, than perform feats of physical labor. Think about that.

Where is your energy heading, while concentrating on one particular issue? Over or under stimulation of vital energy centers brings about disorder in the concentrated energy core. Disease thus unravels through the central nervous system, the endocrine system: the great system that transmits emotional energy into the blood (Blood boiling, cold blooded, etc.)

Mind, body, and soul of man are linked by these supersensible connections. These energy centers harmonize the flow of blood. Emotions serve as the catalyst for humans' evolution, as sense perception has formed man through the ego's design.

This is why emotion will always exist on a certain frequency of conscientiousness. Thoughts are therefore connected with our own organs. Organs are connected to glands and the glands are run by the energy center (chakra). This is a way of linking certain disorders with certain energy centers. Thus if there is over or under activity of a center, conflict and deformity will ensue.

There are seven main energy centers within a human's etheric and physical structure. These focal points serve as hubs for emotional/spiritual vibrations. They are all equally important for their distinct role. The expression of the soul would be deficient if an imbalance exists within a center.

I will begin by discussing the two lower centers. These lower centers are defined as the Base, or root, center and the Sacral center. The Base center, chakra, is the central internal provider of absolute life. The Sacral center, chakra, too is imperative for health as it transmits the procreative desire nature, as well as the lower impulses brought on by the ego's carnal desires. This Sacral Center, conversely, has a great potency and can give birth to our spiritual re-awakening. Our needs are the results of varying impulses. The survival impulse originates in the root chakra. The motion of emotion within the physique also originates in these lower centers, as the animal impulse is constant. Emotional attitudes toward the attainment of external gratification evolve over stages of development. Through these desire vibrations we produce, each soul expresses the illumination of its own soul/astral/karmic/etheric body-whatever you choose to call it. The physical develops with its soul's evolution.

Hitherto, our emotions have formed a desire body that is incorporated with both our etheric body and soul. Some would argue that a pleasure body is accompanied by a pain body. When our astral/etheric body detaches from the physical body and enters into the astral plane, sensory skills no longer exist in this dimension. Pure emotion at certain elemental frequencies is all that now fuels the astral body at this stage of spiritual growth. Therefore, the desire/emotional/karmic body is formed through experience on earth in each lifetime. Disintegration of the emotional experience occurs in accordance with the soul's crystallization.

In a higher frequency the lower centers reach a spiritual sense of wholeness, completion. The lower the vibration the more we are geared toward our lower animal nature. That being said, the base of the spine, the seat of the lower self, is in close proximity with the procreative forces. Therefore, the indescribable super sensible impulses of the soul are corrupted when received by the animal ego. The emotional force is driven by the ego. How is one to transcend the temptations vibrating within the sacral center? Compromising with great forces within the physique, along with receiving external impulses appropriately, is a start- Meditate! The elimination of balanced energy conduction forms dysfunction in the harmony of the finer instruments, such as the nerves and organs. The organs within the jurisdiction of the disordered center are the first to alter.

Thus the mind holds the key! The animal instinct can mutate into a work of fine art. Disavowal of the self's cravings is the beginning of the end for misdirected energy. If the reader is able to accept the suggestion that the world does not revolve around the accomplishment of his/her wants and desires, then the bridge for a higher consciousness may be discovered. Rather the human body serves as a microcosm of the universe we live in- seven planets, seven centers. Each center therefore serves as a planet within the structure of man, with the result being proper magnetic pull and radiation. To understand the design of the etheric body one must understand the purpose of each center.

Some consider the center located in the gut the second brain, or it may be called the solar plexus center. This energy center forms the perception of self, in which a cycle of emotional impulses runs through this chakra. Any instant judgment is formed in the mind this center disrupts its equilibrium. To replenish this center the individual must begin to connect with their divine purpose- a purpose comparable to that of the Sun's etheric body. Some may argue the universal consciousness is still in this stage of recognition of soul.

Ironically, the center above the solar plexus is the heart center- The home for love. A center we must all begin to truly recognize and grasp. It is the one center that rhythmically retains the impulse of infinite unconditional love. There are many definitions for this one eternal trait that will's man to overcome great impassible obstacles. Thus true love is impossible as long as the heart center is disordered and begins to harden.

The throat center is the home of creative divinity. The bestowed wisdom of the higher invisible elemental rays is clearly evident through the higher consciousness of this center. Addiction is a result of dysfunction within this center, an argument that can be made for disorder in any of the center's. Thus, it may begin to become clear how the upper centers can be manipulated from their equilibrium in order to fill the soul's sensations presented to the ego. A misinterpretation of the soul's purpose unfolds externally. Thus if the soul's will is not performing in accordance with divine laws than the creative genius is not connected with divine thought. Creativity is performed for the ego. Thus for many, desires take charge and eliminate the soul's innovative desire to employ change in order to align the macro-soul with the micro-soul. Humanics in action!

Now with so much talk of soul-consciousness we will work up to the centers connected with the mind. The Ajna center sits right between the eyes and it is called the great source of intuition and imagination. The pineal gland's spiritual sense is the doorway into the etheric body.

The last center to mention is the crown center. The Crown is found around the very top of the head. The soul's antenna! But in order for this device to form and run properly- - a change of direction in thought must occur. If a change develops in support of natural growth and budding flowers, the mind will begin to receive the impulses from a higher consciousness. Subtle changes in thinking forms an imperceptible pervasive power that changes the way in which our mind collects impulses. Nothing stays constant in the Universe but the Absolute One, thoughts will forever flow through the ether. Thus a simple floating divine thought could ultimately drive an individual to transform his ego. A divine purpose only runs parallel with pure thoughts.

To surely remove ego the mind must separate three individual forces within the mind. Will, feeling, and thought must be untangled in order for man to find the center within his Ajna center. If this center is recognized the human will soon discover electric currents running through the etheric body. Subtleties ignored in the past now appear as currents within the individual etheric mold. Once the separation is made between thought, feeling, and will in the mind, the next step is to separate the same principles, throughout the body. Therefore a more defined energy vibration begins to develop within the mind. The mind will begin to pay homage to the soul. This mindset will soon present the powerful innocence and reverence held by the infinite soul. Its omnipresence becomes a dominating constant. Thus a soul body illuminates around the etheric and physical vehicle.

Divine thought in the human mind is all manufactured by the invisible elements emitted through the suns invisible rays. Rays pushed forth by the great force of the energy manifestation within the sun are also available for human's benefit through a mental transmutation. We no longer are absorbing or releasing energy that hinders natural growth. Death and decay are qualities we recognize, but do not associate with. Rebirth, renewal, and springtime buds, are all qualities familiar to the spirit of natural well-being. Living with the seasons.

We are no longer a micro-planet, but now we too are a sun emitting rays to benefit the entirety of the universe, with not one thought for self. The increasing vision of natural growth within the permanence of the all-pervading etheric rays will always attract my devotion.

It is true- the mental and chemical pollution we emit is purified by the suns rays and various dimensions. As we relinquish the poisonous toxins through various means (breathing, sweating), the particle matter performs a metamorphous. The physical body is forever developing. The etheric and soul body also undergo changes- with greatest of intensity at the time of death. Truly, death is a time we should most celebrate. It is the soul's return ascent home, shedding the Astral body along the journey.

Our individual Astral body is a microcosm of the greater universal Astral Plane, which some would define as the Ether. Even in physical death, our invisible bodies survive in this Astral Plane. The astral body, following death, begins to call the Astral Plane home. Yes, spirits live within the seven main elements that compose the ether. These seven elements are also widely known as the seven rays.

Spirits and living impulses survive within the elemental ray they are attracted to- The Law of Attraction. There is no equilibrium or neutral within this Astral Plane- high or low, angry or sad. With the mineral content existing in the ether, the connection is made in the physical body with these forces through the magnetic pull of our mind's impulses.

Again, disorder occurs in whichever of the centers that is over-stimulated at the time of thought. Thus we live with and breathe in the invisible dead astral thought carcasses of the past. One thing must be expressed again, there are good and bad rays that are received. It all must be balanced. The nature of the etheric elemental ray absorbed is therefore attracted by the cyclical mental activity.

A ray therefore becomes improper as its frequency enters a realm in which it doesn't connect. In order to grasp the nature of the seven rays we must first grasp all of their qualities. Qualities we can trace back to the sun's form. The rays reflect the seven fulfillments from the "seven Spirits before the throne of God"[i].

The sun is not an elemental ray, but what forms its cosmic force and emitting energies is all the result of the seven elemental God rays. With acceptance that the sun's rays are driven by seven essential rays, we can begin to understand the absolute reality. Through the cycle of time the space has hitherto filled with cosmic rays that develop universal logic, as well as the rays that promote the physical vegetable and animal kingdoms.

Thus the invisible force of the absolute one manifests into concrete external form. This force is active in every life form, even in the invisible nature spirits that make up Earth's etheric body. This being said, there is a great difference between human and animal nature (at times). Humans have the ability to advance their mind, animals, more or less, are stuck in their station. Hence, higher knowledge is continually available in order to develop the mind into an instrument comparable to no other. It is, however, all in the individual's hands to decide whether to follow their own divine purpose or not.

It is the transmitting impulses from the emitting rays in the astral plane which structure vast traits. Research into the rays' powers would be an infinite task no doubt. The first three rays I will define, by legendary Alice A. Bailey, are "The Great Rays of Aspect". She believed consciousness could be separated into three individual categories by these three rays. The ray emitting red conducts the impulse of will and power. The blue ray emits love and emotions. The yellow ray emits intelligence in thought.

These three supersensible rays bridge the gap between the concrete mind and the logic of the gods. These attributes are also necessary for the destiny of the present. All rays are constantly aligned to serve their divine purpose. We must connect! The next four rays will also be described through the color they emit.

These rays are considered those of "attribute". For one developed in color sensory, I have read somewhere that the lighter the shade envisioned the calmer the potency. The rays have polarizing effects.

The orange ray is considered the ray of harmony through conflict. The green rays emit the knowledge of science and concrete physical fact. The purple ray emits devotion and idealism into an energy center. The concluding indigo ray provides the impulse for order and ceremonial magic. Thus, these rays influence energy centers through the energy within the astral plane.

Within the Astral plane, four branches of nature have unraveled through this spirit of the cosmic rays. The mineral kingdom, the vegetable kingdom, the animal kingdom, and the human kingdom all could somewhat define the evolution of nature.

The mineral kingdom deserves essential praise for our development because of the extremes of static activity produced from mineral form- lifeless nature, on one side of the spectrum, and intensity of radiation on the other. Radioactivity results from the mineral attachment to the atomic ether.

Next, the vegetable kingdom is grounded within the soil of the earth. We must keep in mind that whatever composes the soil, will compose the plant. This kingdom may provide a prime example of disorder within an energy center. Is the food you're eating natural?

Are man's acts driven by materialistic cravings depleting the equilibrium of the earth's purpose?

Thirdly, the animal kingdom, just as all kingdoms, is ever evolving. The development of instinct and intuition enable man to be the king of this category. It is in his liberation from this lower self that man will promote himself into the human kingdom.

The human kingdom we could still consider undeveloped as it has not fully emerged. This is the kingdom where the higher elements connect with the device in the head that only could become developed through divine intent. "What stands above, sits below." Thus liberation from the thoughts triggered by external forms allow one to begin to understand the emotional energy fueling the macrocosm.

The mind's development is similar as to that which unfolds within the mineral kingdom. The depths and dimensions reached during the crystallization of a mineral also unfold within man's mind. Hence, if one develops the mind to such a fine gold impulse, one will emit a golden aura. Is this mind transmutation already determined within the evolutionary rings of the universe? Or is it a race against time to repair our destruction?

There are evolutionary stages within the life cycle of a mineral, in which their forms could be divided into three sections- baser metals, standard metals, and semiprecious stones. Now what if human activity is altering the mineral structure of the ether?

Is manmade particle matter disrupting the ether provided by the heavens? Is there too much pollution for the rays to purify? Are the rays so severely polluted that our individual etheric centers are dysfunctioning as a result?

Destruction of nature may reflect the same deadly destructive power capable of removing our etheric form from our physical. Thus, it is of my greatest interest if it is possible for earth's physical form to break from its etheric body, just as a dying carcass breaks ties with the etheric and soul body. Is the earth withstanding such a great destructive disorder?

Some argue that humans have created the condition of the Earth. What if the fate of the world now lies in our hands. We continually drain the recourses out of the earth. Can the earth sustain itself through such rapid depletion? We are also adding tons of waste into the earth as well. Maybe we can passionately change all this. All we have done is take, take, take, we never have given back. The Earth needs a whole lot of unconditional love! What if it is possible to strengthen the earth. What if I told you microscopic bugs may be our solution. Micro-organisms are essential to soil composition and health. There are little parasites dancing around your body as you read.

Soil depletion is a great ill cast upon the earth. *Indefinable Spirits* live in the earth, in the plant, in the evaporating water, in the gases, in the air, in the heavens, all of which are essential to plant and human growth. What if those spirits are vastly depleted? Can they be restored?

Soil replenishment is where we should maybe begin to look- improved consistency. The extraction and absorption of cosmic, solar, and earthly forces at a greater magnetic attraction may portray the ability to rejuvenate and repair our earth. It must all be driven by spiritual ego nevertheless. This Divine Will for change can repair our de-energized food and repair ourselves within.

The most important thing I hope the reader takes from this work is that it is possible to fix yourself by first simply examining your soul. A simple task of correcting the flow of the spirit is a beginning. Sound health therefore develops in the mind rather than the physique. Now if the energies begin to change flow in order to repair our individual disorders, then maybe the energetic dysfunction we feed the ether will subside.

Some consider a portion of the natural spirits as ever changing microscopic parasites. This ever changing form is a clear indication as to why brain matter evolves. In "What is Biodynamics", Rudolf Steiner claims, "The human brain is the evolved product of elimination." What if there is no longer any beneficial natural spirits in our food? In a sense our food is depleted of nutrition to appease capital gain. What is a fruits value? The value of a fruit should not rest in its material impression, but rather in the composition of the elements that formed the material. There is a certain vitality in play that is necessary for both spiritual and plant growth.

It seems to me that vast unlimited energies have been spent on the analysis of a disease. What about the cure? Rather than make the effect the focal point, why not investigate and study the individual, as that, an individual. The causes and symptoms need to be traced back to its energy provider.

In conclusion, if there's a will, there's a way! We can accomplish anything, but we must first change within. We must unite ourselves with what is truly living, seen or unseen. It is now time to promote both the individual and universal well-being! Earth is in the process of dying, we need to heal it, and heal it now! Remember, soil with humus like substances in the process of decomposition contains living ether, and it is the soil that ultimately becomes the plant's mask.

Think of how we feed the earth in so many negative ways, non-disposable garbage, synthetics, dead carcasses filled with disease, water-soluble fertilizers. Yes, have you ever thought of the earth filled with dead decaying diseased carcasses? Cremation serves so many wonderful purposes. It keeps a body from taking up a nice sized plot. Fire kills the disease still vital inside the dead carcass as well. Cremation also sends the astral body into the astral plane much quicker than that of the burial of what remains.

What happens to the invisible elements that formed the mind, the emotions, the soul, the astral body? Dissolution of the Astral body occurs through cycles of reincarnation. The soul's break from the karmic emotional body is a gradual process through the law of attraction.

The harmonizing of a disordered impulse within the physical state ascends the elemental ray from the astral body back to the correlating universal element making up the celestial. Human Beings are the only form that hold the rare ability to repair disorder above within the heavens. Thus, the damaged soul purifies itself by removing the desire impulses of the astral plane from its body. Finally, the soul reaches home.

So remember, in order to fix within, start with what you feed it, both in thought and food. Food becomes poison for the lower senses, as nourishment is found in toxic preservatives bound for the intestines, the great storage unit of the toxins. Henceforth, if you have a quarter acre you can still plant or enrich some stuff. You can grow some food, you can enrich the soil. You can even enrich your soul by reading a good book under a beautiful tree!

I will close in the words of Rudolf Steiner, "Anything raised above the normal level for that locale will show a particular tendency to life, a propensity to become permeated with etheric vitality."

---

[1] The Seven Rays of Life, Alice A. Bailey